MW01100250

food user manual

Ryan Bradley, ND, MPH & Sonja Max, MS, RD

©2012, 2013 by Ryan Bradley, ND, MPH and Sonja Max, MS, RD

All rights reserved. No part of this book may be reproduced in any form or by any electronic or mechanical means, including information storage and retrieval systems, without permission in writing from the authors, except brief passages quoted for the purposes of a review.

ISBN 978-0-9849408-0-6

Created by Ryan Bradley, ND, MPH and Sonja Max, MS, RD
order online: **www.foodusermanual.com** | email: info@foodusermanual.com

♲ Printed on recycled paper

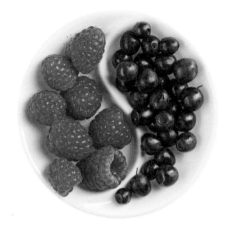

Table of contents

Symbols used in this manual:

☺ enjoy often

☺ eat in moderation

😐 eat occasionally, if at all

☹ avoid or minimize

What's so bad about fat?

Nothing, but there are important facts to know. Fat is found in almost every food we eat. There are many different kinds of fats. Fats are used for energy or stored in tissues when too much is consumed. Some fats are used for brain function, vision and healthy skin. Other fats can lead to high cholesterol, triglycerides and many preventable diseases, including atherosclerosis.

Fats provide 9 calories of energy per gram (compared to 4 calories per gram of protein or carbohydrates). One tablespoon of ANY fat or oil provides 120 calories.

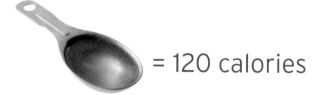 = 120 calories

Know your fatty acids.

🙂 Omega-3: Cold-water fish, flax seeds, chia seeds, walnuts

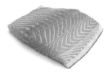

🙂 Polyunsaturated & monounsaturated: Nuts, seeds, avocado, olive oil, vegetable oils

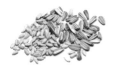

😐 Saturated: Cheese, milk, butter, red meat, poultry, coconut oil, palm oil

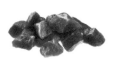

☹️ Hydrogenated oil, trans fats: Margarine, shortening, crackers, cookies, cakes, prepared foods, fried foods

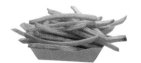
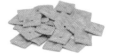

How much do I need?

The World Health Organization recommends:

Minimum calories from fat: 15% (men) 20% (women)

Maximum calories from fat: 30-35% (men & women)

Research suggests that **halting and/or reversing heart disease** through diet requires:

Following a plant-based diet with few or no added oils. Necessary fats in this diet come from nuts and seeds, with a small amount from beans, whole grains and vegetables.[1,2]

The DASH eating plan (Dietary Approaches to Stop Hypertension) recommends the following for someone on a 2,000 calorie diet (if your calorie needs are less, reduce accordingly):

Fat Source:	Number of Servings:
Low fat or non fat dairy foods	2 - 4 per day
Lean meats, fish, poultry	2 or less per day
Nuts, seeds, and legumes	4 - 5 per week
Fats and sweets	Limited

Bottom Line: Decide how much you wish to reduce your heart disease risk and manage your weight. Eat accordingly. Ask your naturopathic doctor, dietitian or integrative medicine practitioner how much and which kind(s) of fat are appropriate for your goals, including specific calorie needs for weight maintenance.

What does it all mean?

Fat is important and essential to include in your diet. Choose plant-based foods and fish. They provide all the essential fats, protein, vitamins and minerals you need to stay heart healthy. Here's an example:

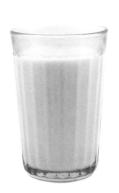

vs.

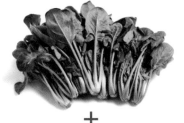

+

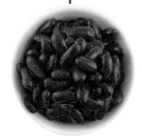

Puzzled by labels?

8 oz. 2% Milk		1/3 cup Black Beans + 1 cup Steamed Spinach	
Calories:	122	Calories:	117
Cal from fat:	43 (35% fat)	Cal from fat:	3 (3% fat)
Protein	8 grams	Protein	10 grams
Calcium	29% RDA	Calcium	25% RDA
Iron	0% RDA	Iron	42% RDA
Fiber	0% RDA	Fiber	56% RDA

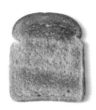

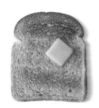

Whole Grain Toast

Calories:	69
Cal from fat:	**10 (14% fat)**

Whole Grain Toast
+ 1 Butter Pat

Calories:	105
Cal from fat:	**46 (44% fat)**

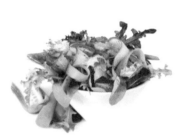

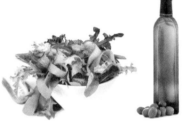

Giant Salad

Calories:	~40
Cal from fat:	**1 (2% fat)**

Giant Salad
+ 1 Tablespoon Oil in Dressing

Calories:	~160
Cal from fat:	**121 (75% fat)**

Puzzled by labels?

Reading labels to find out **how many total calories** in a
serving and **how many calories come from fat** is a much
better guide than looking at **grams** of fat per serving.
(Calories from fat / total calories) x (100) = percent fat

What does research say?

Aggressive plant-based diets may be as effective at lowering cholesterol levels as statin drugs.[3] These diets include functional compounds such as plant sterols, viscous fibers, soy products and almonds, which have been shown to reduce LDL cholesterol.[3,4]

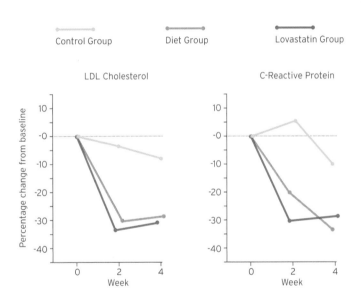

Control Group   Diet Group   Lovastatin Group

The above results, published in 2003 by JAMA, illustrate that the cholesterol-lowering effect of a low-fat plant-based diet with added functional foods is not significantly different from the drug Lovastatin in hyperlipidemic adults.[3] Inflammation was also reduced on this protocol, as measured by C-reactive protein.

Carbo-what?

Carbohydrates are found in starchy and sweet foods. They are not evil. They should not be eliminated from your diet. They are the only source of fuel that your brain uses on a daily basis. Your muscles use them when you exercise but store them as fat when they are not burned for energy. Thus, intake should ideally be proportional to physical activity levels.

Just like fats, they come in many varieties. The more your food looks like the plant from which it came, the healthier it is for you. That means a bowl of wheat berries is healthier than a biscuit. What's a wheat berry? Read on.

What is a refined grain?

🙂 Wheat berries, brown rice, barley, quinoa, oats: These whole grains produce a little package containing carbohydrates, protein and a small amount of healthy fat along with fiber, vitamins and minerals. **Unrefined**, they are edible in their whole, or natural state, and among the most nutritious foods on earth.

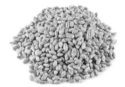 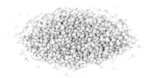

🙂 Whole grain flours: The whole grain is ground into a fine powder. Most of the fiber, vitamins and minerals remain. Look for "100% whole grain" on breads, cereals and pastas.

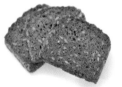

☹ White rice, white flours: The outer, brown coating has been tumbled off. This removes the fiber, the healthy fats, some protein and nearly all of the vitamins and minerals. **Refined** flour makes up white bread, muffins, crackers, cereals, cookies, pastries, pasta, and other "processed" foods.

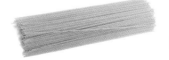 

Carbs and blood sugar

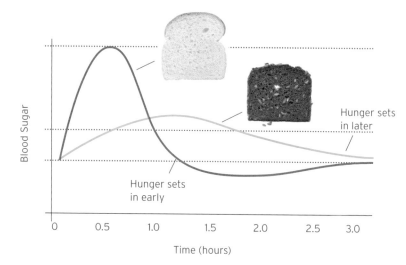

Blood sugar rises slowly and falls slowly (green line) after whole grains are eaten. The fiber in these foods is digested very slowly, allowing gradual release and breakdown of the sugars.

Blood sugar rises quickly (red line) after refined carbohydrates are consumed. This includes juice, soda, refined grains, corn syrup and sugar. Why? Because there is no fiber left in the food to slow digestion! These foods have a **high glycemic index**.

In the red line case, a lot of **insulin** is released to lower blood sugar quickly. This much insulin can cause blood sugar to drop below normal, initiating hunger signals. Ever feel hungry after a large meal when you think you should feel full? This is why!

Balanced meals & snacks

A diet high in refined carbohydrates over many years can lead to **reduced insulin sensitivity**: when insulin is released, but the cells ignore the signal, so blood sugar stays high. This is quite dangerous and leads to type 2 diabetes over time. It is important to balance meals and snacks with adequate protein, fat and fiber, and to exercise often to stay sensitive (to insulin!).

For optimal health, refined grains with a high glycemic index should be minimized or avoided all together. However, other healthy dietary components may help reduce their bad effects. Research has shown that adding a small quantity of nuts to these foods can lower glycemic response.[5,6,7,8]

Tips for reducing glycemic response:

• Adding 60 grams (~1/3 cup) of **almonds** to a breakfast of orange juice and Cream of Wheat® significantly lowered participants' glycemic response, not just for breakfast, but for lunch as well! The addition of almonds also increased satiety throughout the day. [5]

• Healthy participants consumed a glass of juice and a bagel, either with 20 grams of butter or 25 grams of **peanut butter**. Glycemic response was 54% lower after eating the peanut butter snack than the plain butter snack.[6]

• Adding **pistachios** to either white bread, white rice, pasta or potatoes has been shown to lower their glycemic response. [7]

But they look like birdseed!

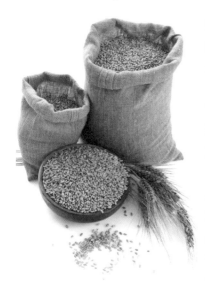

It's true. But they are also much less expensive than meat and dairy products.

They can usually be purchased in bulk at your local supermarket, and cooked easily.

And with the right spices and a little time, your taste buds will actually enjoy the rich, nutty flavors of whole grains. Try these easy grains first:

Quinoa: This whole grain is a complete protein, native to South America. Place 1/2 cup quinoa and 1 cup water into a saucepan with a handful of raisins, 1/2 teaspoon curry powder, 1/2 teaspoon chili powder, and cover. Bring to a boil, turn down heat, and let simmer 15-20 minutes (or until all the liquid is absorbed and the grain is translucent with little tails). Serve with greens and garnish with chopped cilantro and pumpkin seeds.

TIP: Place a handful or two of chopped broccoli or cauliflower on top of the quinoa 5 minutes before it is done cooking and replace lid. The vegetables will gently steam on top of the grain.

Buckwheat: Buckwheat is also considered a complete protein source. For a hearty breakfast, try a creamy buckwheat cereal. Add some raisins and cinnamon, and cook according to directions. Top with ground flaxseeds, chopped walnuts and fresh or frozen (thawed) berries.

TIP: Steel cut oats can be prepared similarly. To shorten cooking time, soak in the cooking water the night before.

Don't be fooled! Strawberries and cream flavored instant oats have 12 times as much sugar, half the fiber and over twice the sodium of plain oats, and not a single strawberry or ounce of cream. What would this do to your blood glucose levels?

Puzzled by labels?

Thick Oats (1/2 cup dry)		Quick Oats (1 pack)		Flavored Oats (1 pack)	
Calories	150	Calories	100	Calories	130
Fiber	4 g	Fiber	3 g	Fiber	2 g
Sodium	0 mg	Sodium	75 mg	Sodium	180 mg
Sugars	1 g	Sugars	1 g	Sugars	12 g

Protein

Protein is found in a variety of foods. Meat, eggs, dairy, nuts, seeds, beans, rice, quinoa, and even broccoli contain protein. Long chains of smaller nutrients called amino acids make up each protein. A nutritionally complete protein includes 9 "essential" amino acids that the body needs in order to maintain healthy hair, skin, nails, muscles and many other tissues.

Animal foods contain all 9 essential amino acids. Plant foods may be lacking one or two essential amino acids. However, by combining a variety of plant foods (grains together with beans or legumes), it is easy to obtain complete sources of protein.

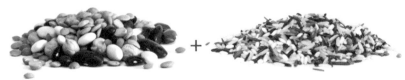

= Complete protein

How much do I need?

The American Dietetic Association recommends 0.8 grams of protein per kilogram of body weight (g/kg) for healthy individuals. Thus, for a 180-pound person: 180 ÷ 2.2 = 81.8 kg. 81.8 kg x 0.8 g/kg = 65.5 grams protein. If protein is divided evenly throughout 3 meals in a day, how much protein is this per meal?

Most Americans consume much more protein than they need, especially at dinner. Protein content of some foods is listed below. Which ones are healthier? Turn the page!

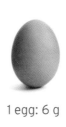

1 egg: 6 g

8 oz. milk: 8 g

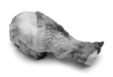

3 oz. chicken: 27 g

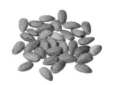

1/4 c almonds: 7 g

1 c quinoa: 8 g

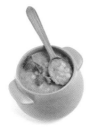

1 c lentils: 18 g

Choose wisely

Getting the right amount protein is important. Equally important, are the other nutrients found **together with** the protein in
any given food.

☺ Plant proteins: Unprocessed beans, whole grains, nuts,
seeds and vegetables provide protein along with healthy
fats, fiber, vitamins, minerals and extra goodies like antioxidants or compounds that help prevent cancer and heart
disease. Plant foods never contain cholesterol. Some actually
contain cholesterol-lowering "phytosterols!"

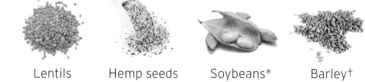

Lentils   Hemp seeds   Soybeans*   Barley†

☺ Functional proteins: Yogurt, fish and whey are all good
sources of protein. They contain elements such as probiotics (in yogurt) or omega-3 fatty acids (in cold-water fish)
that are necessary for good health. They do contain some
cholesterol and lack fiber. Choose plain yogurt, and cold-
water fish such as salmon or sardines.

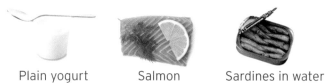

Plain yogurt   Salmon   Sardines in water

*Many soybeans are genetically modified. Look for organic or non-GMO soy.

Should protein found together with saturated fat and cholesterol be thought of differently than protein found with fiber and polyunsaturated fats? You bet!

😐 Eggs, lean poultry, low-fat dairy: Eggs, lean poultry, low-fat cottage cheese and low-fat milk contain protein along with cholesterol and saturated fats. They do not contain fiber. Beware: 2% milk (by weight) is actually 35% fat by calories!

| Eggs | Skinless chicken | Cottage cheese |

☹️ High-fat and processed protein: Red meat, pork, fried meats, dark meat poultry, poultry skin, cured ham, bacon, sausage, hot dogs, deli meats, and full-fat dairy all contain high amounts of saturated fat. Additionally, they may contain excess salt, require frying oil or chemicals such as nitrates to extend shelf life and maintain color. These foods may increase risk of heart disease and diabetes and should be avoided.

| Salami | Deli meat | Smoked meat | Cheese |

†Barley, wheat, spelt, kamut and rye contain a protein called "gluten." Ask your ND, RD or integrative medicine MD if you think you may be intolerant to gluten.

Not enough protein?

Research indicates that too little protein, or a ratio too high in carbohydrates and too low in protein, can lead to weight gain and decreased lean muscle mass.[9]

Simple carbohydrate cravings or **sugar cravings** are often a sign of too little protein intake.

"Balanced daily distribution of protein with increased intake at breakfast and lunch protects metabolically active tissues including skeletal muscle during weight loss." [9]

-Suzanne Devkota & Donald K. Layman

Have protein at breakfast: For a daily protein requirement of 72 grams (body weight 200 pounds), 24 grams of protein is needed at breakfast, lunch and dinner! The following breakfast contains 24 grams of protein:

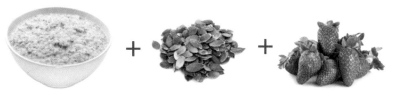

1/2 cup (dry) creamy buckwheat cereal (10 g protein)	2 oz. (1/4 cup) pumpkin seeds (14 g protein)	1/2 cup fresh berries (<1 g protein)

Protein and blood sugar

Researchers have demonstrated that a high-protein snack **two hours before breakfast** leads to reduced glycemic response after breakfast. Response was measured as total blood sugar over time, which was reduced by 40% when the high-protein snack was consumed.[10] The snack consisted of 30 grams of soy nuts and 75 grams of yogurt. Could this be added to your routine?

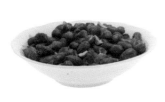 +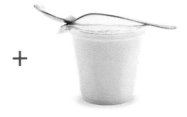

30 g soy nuts
(~1/8 cup or 2 tablespoons)
13 g protein

75 g yogurt (plain)
(~1/2 cup)
4 g protein

Animal or plant protein?

A Dutch study followed 38,094 participants for 10 years to determine how protein intake affects risk for developing diabetes. Increased risk for diabetes was associated with higher overall protein intake and higher animal protein intake. Vegetable protein intake was not associated with higher risk for diabetes.[11]

Hydrate...

...or die! What to drink can be just as confusing as what to eat. With hundreds of options in the beverage aisle, how is one supposed to know what's best?

The short answer: **water is best.** It is usually free. It is nature's perfect thirst quencher. It has no calories, no sugar and no harmful artificial ingredients. Each cell in the body is designed to function efficiently in the presence of water. Often people find they have more energy when they increase their water intake.

The longer answer: If you absolutely need flavor, choose beverages that are natural and unsweetened, and very low in sugar (read labels). See the next page for guidance on selecting healthier drinks.

When water just won't do:

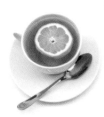

☺ Natural and calorie-free: Try herbal teas or green tea (brewed at home); sparkling mineral water; or water with a slice of lemon or lime. Aim for zero calories when reading labels. Sweeteners such as stevia and xylitol are acceptable.

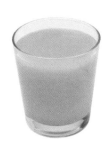

☺ 100% fruit juice: Fruit juice contains more natural vitamins and antioxidants than soda and other empty-calorie beverages. However, note the calories and the high glycemic index! A whole apple has more fiber, more nutrients and fewer calories than a 10 ounce glass of apple juice. A carrot and a glass of water contain more electrolytes than a sports drink and are less expensive. Try to eat your fruit instead of drinking it.

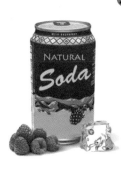

☹ Soda and flavored coffee drinks: High-calorie, sugary beverages taste good, but are addictive and cause weight gain. Flavored coffee drinks can contain upwards of 400 calories and 80 grams of sugar! Whether they are sweetened with real sugar or high fructose corn syrup, there is no need for these beverages in a healthy diet.

Sugar content comparison

There are 4.2 grams of sugar in one teaspoon. A 12-ounce soda contains approximately 10.7 teaspoons – or a quarter cup – of sugar. This equates to 180 calories of sugar.

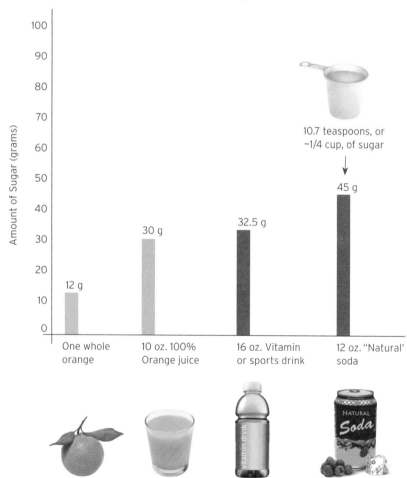

Amount of Sugar (grams)

10.7 teaspoons, or ~1/4 cup, of sugar

12 g	30 g	32.5 g	45 g
One whole orange	10 oz. 100% Orange juice	16 oz. Vitamin or sports drink	12 oz. "Natural" soda

Alcohol: Alcohol contains 7 calories per gram, whereas protein and carbohydrates contain 4 calories per gram. Alcohol can cause weight gain as well as liver damage. Discuss individual alcohol intake with your naturopathic doctor, dietitian or integrative medicine practitioner.

Diet soda: Diet soda has no calories or real sugar. However, research shows that "tricking" the body with a sweet taste on the tongue, without following through on calories, may cause an increase in appetite as well as weight gain.[12]

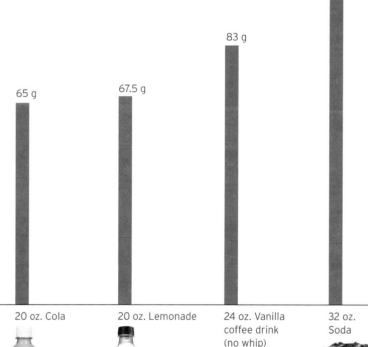

| 65 g | 67.5 g | 83 g | 104 g |
| 20 oz. Cola | 20 oz. Lemonade | 24 oz. Vanilla coffee drink (no whip) | 32 oz. Soda |

Other Nutrients

So far we have discussed "macronutrients," or fat, carbohydrates and proteins, which all provide calories. "Micronutrients," which do not provide calories, are also necessary for optimal health and disease prevention. These include:

- Vitamins
- Minerals
- Bioactive compounds such as:
  - Phenols
  - Carotenoids
  - Lignans
  - Plant sterols & stanols
  - Probiotics
  - Organosulfur compounds

Nutrient density

Foods that are more "nutrient dense" have more micronutrients per calorie. They may be eaten in greater quantities, with few adverse effects. Would one ounce of steak fill you up? How about 2 cups of broccoli? If you tend to overeat, fill up on low-calorie, nutrient dense plant foods for a variety of healthy vitamins, minerals and bioactive compounds.

Puzzled by labels?

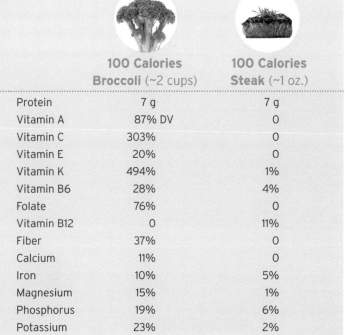

	100 Calories Broccoli (~2 cups)	100 Calories Steak (~1 oz.)
Protein	7 g	7 g
Vitamin A	87% DV	0
Vitamin C	303%	0
Vitamin E	20%	0
Vitamin K	494%	1%
Vitamin B6	28%	4%
Folate	76%	0
Vitamin B12	0	11%
Fiber	37%	0
Calcium	11%	0
Iron	10%	5%
Magnesium	15%	1%
Phosphorus	19%	6%
Potassium	23%	2%

Spare the salt

A deficiency or excess of a particular vitamin or mineral may be damaging to our health. Two minerals of concern are sodium and potassium.

Sodium and potassium work together to maintain fluid balance throughout cells in the body. They are also important for proper nerve function and muscle control.

Consuming too much sodium and not enough potassium increases risk of high blood pressure, stroke, kidney stones and osteoporosis. Americans usually eat far too much sodium and not nearly enough potassium. See the comparison below:

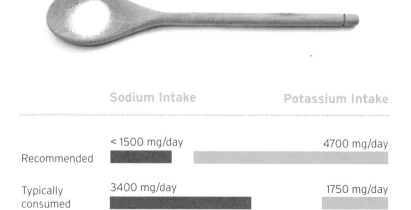

	Sodium Intake	Potassium Intake
Recommended	< 1500 mg/day	4700 mg/day
Typically consumed	3400 mg/day	1750 mg/day

Foods in bags, boxes, cans and wrappers are usually high in sodium. Foods packaged by nature are usually not.

	Sodium (per 100 g serving)	Potassium
Beef jerky	2790 mg	235 mg
Ramen soup	2002 mg	185 mg
Italian dressing	1759 mg	231 mg
Parmesan Cheese	1630 mg	29 mg
Glazed chicken	1529 mg	125 mg
Pancake mix	1438 mg	329 mg
Kale	70 mg	450 mg
Flaxseeds	30 mg	813 mg
Yams	9 mg	816 mg
Pistachio nuts (unsalted)	10 mg	1042 mg
White beans (dried)	16 mg	1795 mg
Dried parsley	452 mg	3805 mg

Not in your multivitamin!

Emerging research suggests that bioactive compounds have extremely important health benefits. Plant foods such as onions, garlic, root vegetables, berries, fruits, specialty mushrooms, nuts, seeds, leafy green vegetables, broccoli, soy beans, green tea and avocados all contain these compounds. Some bioactive compounds act as "antioxidants," (see p. 30) to help counteract oxidative damage done by free radicals.

Fiber
Cholesterol-lowering, improves intestinal health

Apigenin
Antioxidant, anti-inflammatory and anti-cancer properties[13]

Ferulic acid
Antioxidant, anti-inflammatory, anti-diabetic[14], protects against Alzheimer's disease[15]

Carnitine
Essential for converting fatty acids into energy

β-sitosterol
Cholesterol-lowering, anti-inflammatory[16] anti-cancer properties[17, 18]

Other bioactive compounds may lower cholesterol, improve cell metabolism or prevent cancer. The figure below shows just a few compounds in green vegetables. More are discovered every day! Many of these little goodies are lost in processing or cooking. What's in an orange may not be in orange juice, and is definitely not in orange soda. This is true for most foods. They are most nutritious when eaten fresh, whole and unprocessed.

Betalains
Protect against oxidative and nitrosative stress[19]

Lutein
Decreases risk of age-related macular degeneration, anti-tumor properties[20]

Quercetin
Antihypertensive, lowers oxidized LDL[21]

Furfuran-type lignans
Anti-cancer, antioxidant, cardioprotective, neuroprotective, anti-inflammatory properties[22]

Glucosinolates
Aid in detoxification, anti-cancer properties, Anti-inflammatory[23, 24, 25]

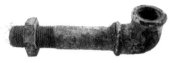

Be flexible… in your arteries

Poor dietary choices can cause immediate damage to blood vessels due to an increase in "free radicals" and oxidative damage. Simply put, arteries can become corroded pipes, which no longer deliver nutrients and oxygen where they are needed. Restricting sugary foods and carefully selecting fats can prevent this corrosion. "Polyphenols" found in foods have also been shown to prevent damage.

Ellagic acid in raspberries has been shown to reduce carotid artery wall thickness and reduce blood pressure.

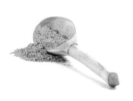

Tetrahydrocurcumin in turmeric may prevent lipid oxidation caused by free radicals and help reduce cholesterol. It is also known to decrease blood glucose and increase serum insulin levels.

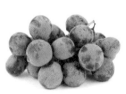

Resveratrol in nuts and the skin of red grapes exhibits antioxidant, antithrombotic, and anti-inflammatory properties, and inhibits carcinogenesis.

Catechins in green tea may also prevent artery damage from free radicals.

Forget the big words

Notice how colorful healthy foods are? A balanced variety of bioactive compounds can be achieved by eating a variety of colors every day. You do not need to learn scientific names or memorize food facts (unless you want to). **Just eat the rainbow.** Daily.

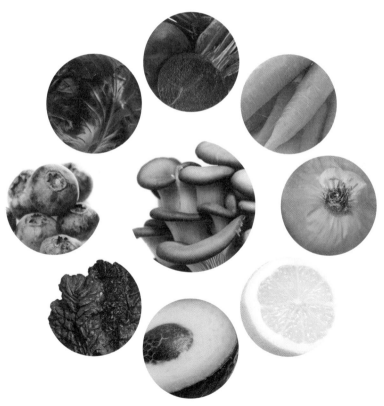

Inflammation

The body uses inflammation naturally to stabilize a condition such as a sprained ankle, a cut, bruise, or an infection. Blood cells and natural chemicals are quickly sent to the site of injury, which can cause swelling, redness or itchiness. This response is necessary for good health.

However, inflammation may also become chronic, or happen over a long period of time in places we might not see or feel as much as a sprained ankle. This can be caused by **poor diet, stress, inadequate sleep or a lack of physical activity**. Chronic, low-grade inflammation of this type contributes to the health consequences of conditions such as atherosclerosis, rheumatoid arthritis, obesity and type 2 diabetes. Why not do what you can to reduce inflammation by eating a healthy diet and treating your body well?

How does it happen?

Meals high in sugar, animal fat and "advanced glycation end products" are just a few dietary sources of inflammation. Call them AGEs for short (and yes, they will make you age!). These can form on foods during cooking, or inside the body from metabolic processes. When foods are grilled or heated to high temperatures, they form AGEs, usually seen by blackening or browning.

Blackening of grilled meats or vegetables

Browning of potatoes and starchy foods

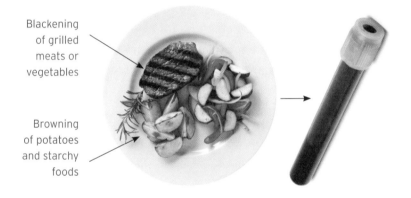

The European Journal of Nutrition reported that people with diabetes who have a high intake of dietary AGEs had significantly higher levels of Hemoglobin A1c, LDL cholesterol and AGEs in the blood compared to diabetics with low AGE intake or healthy controls. High AGE intake subjects also had higher levels of inflammation (measured by 8-isoprostane, IL-1α) and lower antioxidant activity (SOD).[26] Evidence is accumulating that AGEs may contribute to diabetic neuropathy (numbness), retinopathy (blindness) and other serious complications.[27]

How do I stop it?

1) Eat a healthy diet. Foods not correlated with an increase in disease include: fresh fruits, raw and steamed or lightly cooked vegetables, whole grains, beans, lentils, nuts, seeds, sea vegetables and many herbs and spices.

2) Include anti-inflammatory foods. Spices such as turmeric and ginger, fresh **herbs** such as basil, cilantro, and parsley, leafy greens, berries and **omega-3 fats** in flax seeds and cold-water fish all have anti-inflammatory properties. Most brightly colored **vegetables** are also anti-inflammatory.

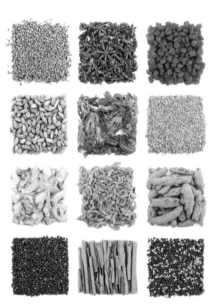

Spices have been used for centuries in cooking throughout Asia, Europe and Latin America. Many spices are known to prevent or reduce oxidative damage of foods during the cooking process. This, in turn, reduces AGEs and other potentially toxic components of cooked foods.

3) Exercise. For optimal health benefits, the Dietary Guidelines for Americans recommends:

"Adults should increase their aerobic physical activity to 300 minutes (5 hours) a week of moderate-intensity, or 150 minutes a week of vigorous-intensity aerobic physical activity, or an equivalent combination of moderate- and vigorous-intensity activity. Additional health benefits are gained by engaging in physical activity beyond this amount. Adults should also include muscle-strengthening activities... on 2 or more days a week." [28]

The effects of exercise only last about 24 hours. It is important to exercise **daily** for optimal benefits.

4) Reduce Stress. Whether it is taking 5-10 slow, deep breaths before each meal, meditating daily or practicing yoga, research has shown that quieting the mind and learning how to consciously respond to stressful situations may reduce inflammation as well as improve cognitive performance.[29,30]

5) Sleep. Poor sleep quality and short duration are associated with increased inflammation.[31] Make your health a priority by eliminating the less important things that keep you from sleeping. Exposure to adequate daylight as well as exercise may also improve sleep quality.

Summing up

Dietary habits are difficult to change. But the more you change at once, the better you will feel and the better your body will perform.

 Distribute your food intake throughout the day. Consume adequate protein in the morning. Try not to eat within a few hours of bedtime.

Consume nutrient-dense, balanced meals and snacks that will not raise your blood sugar rapidly.

Reduce inflammation by eating anti-inflammatory foods, exercising daily, sleeping and reducing stress.

Work with a naturopathic physician, dietitian and/or integrative medicine practitioner for optimal results.

Healthy habit map

Most of the dietary and lifestyle concepts covered in this manual can be summed up in the diagram below. Sleep, water and exercise are central to the health of every body. Whole, unprocessed plant foods are the key to a healthy diet. Added oils, sweets, dairy products, refined foods and meats are optional and do not need to be consumed daily if needs are met with nutrient dense vegetables, legumes and whole grains.

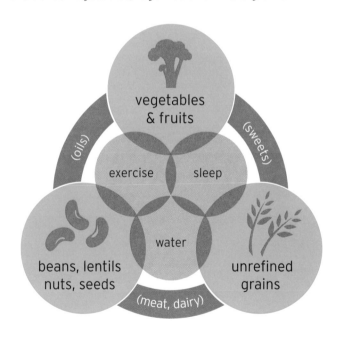

"Eat a healthy diet, with an emphasis on plant sources."

- American Cancer Society

My goals

Daily Servings:	Getting started Visit 1: ___ /___	Raising the bar Visit 2:___ /___	Keeping it high Visit 3:___ /___
Vegetables			
Fruit			
Beans/lentils			
Nuts/seeds			
Whole grains			
Fish			
Water (cups)			
(Dairy)			
(Meat)			
(Sweets)			
Minutes of aerobic exercise			
Minutes of weight-bearing exercise			
Hours of Sleep			

Notes

References

1) Chainani-Wu N, Weidner G, Purnell DM, Frenda S, Merritt-Worden T, Pischke C, Campo R, Kemp C, Kersh ES, Ornish D. Changes in emerging cardiac biomarkers after an intensive lifestyle intervention. *Am J Cardiol* 2011;108(4):498-507.

2) Esselstyn CB Jr. Resolving the Coronary Artery Disease Epidemic Through Plant-Based Nutrition. *Preventive Cardiology* Fall 2001: 171-177

3) Jenkins DJA, Kendall CWC, Marchie A, Faulkner DA, Wong JMW, de Souza R, Emam A, Parker TL; Vidgen E, Lapsley KG, Trautwein EA, Josse RG, Leiter LA, Connelly PW. Effects of a Dietary Portfolio of Cholesterol-Lowering Foods vs Lovastatin on Serum Lipids and C-Reactive Protein *JAMA* 2003;290(4):502-510.

4) Gardner CD, Coulston A, Chatterjee L, Rigby A, Spiller G, Farquhar JW. The Effect of a Plant-Based Diet on Plasma Lipids in Hypercholesterolemic Adults *Ann Intern Med.* 2005;142:725-733

5) Jenkins DJA, Kendall CWC, Josse AR, et al. Almonds decrease postprandial glycemia, insulinemia, and oxidative damage in healthy individuals. *J Nutr* 2006;136:2987-2992

6) Johnston CS, Buller AJ. Vinegar and Peanut Products as Complementary Foods to Reduce Postprandial Glycemia *Journal of the American Dietetic Association* 2005;105(12):1939-1942

7) Mori AM, Considine RV, Mattes RD. Acute and second-meal effects of almond form in impaired glucose tolerant adults: a randomized crossover trial, *Nutrition & Metabolism* 2011; 8:6

8) Kendall CWC, Josse AR, Esfahani A, Jenkins DJA, The impact of pistachio intake alone or in combination with high-carbohydrate foods on post-prandial glycemia, *European Journal of Clinical Nutrition* 65, 696-702, June 2011

9) Devkota S and Layman DK, Protein metabolic roles in treatment of obesity *Current Opinion in Clinical Nutrition and Metabolic Care 2010;* 13:403-407

10) Chen MJ, Jovanovic A, Taylor R, Utilizing the Second-Meal Effect in Type 2 Diabetes: Practical Use of a Soya-Yogurt Snack, *Diabetes Care* 2010;33:2552-2554

11) Sluijs I, Beulens JWJ, Van Der A D, Spijkerman AMW, Grobbee DE, Van Der Schouw, YT, Dietary Intake of Total, Animal, and Vegetable Protein and Risk of Type 2 Diabetes in the European Prospective Investigation into Cancer and Nutrition (EPIC)-NL Study, *Diabetes Care* 2010;33, 43-48

12) Hampton T. Sugar substitutes linked to weight gain. *JAMA* 2008;299(18):2137-8.

13) Shukla S, Gupta S, Apigenin: A Promising Molecule for Cancer Prevention *Pharm Res.* 2010 June; 27(6): 962–978.

14) Choi R, Kim BH, Naowaboot J, Lee MY, Hyun MR, Cho EJ, Lee ES, Lee EY, Yang YC, Chung CH. Effects of ferulic acid on diabetic nephropathy in a rat model of type 2 diabetes. *Exp Mol Med.* 2011 Oct 6. [Epub ahead of print]

15) Pocernich CB, Lange ML, Sultana R, Butterfield DA. Nutritional approaches to modulate oxidative stress in Alzheimer's disease. *Curr Alzheimer Res.* 2011 Aug;8(5):452-69.

16) Othman RA, Moghadasian MH. Beyond cholesterol-lowering effects of plant sterols: clinical and experimental evidence of anti-inflammatory properties. *Nutr Rev.* 2011 Jul;69(7):371-82.

17) Baskar AA, Ignacimuthu S, Paulraj GM, Al Numair KS. Chemopreventive potential of beta-Sitosterol in experimental colon cancer model – an in vitro and In vivo study. *BMC Complement Altern Med.* 2010 Jun 4;10:24.

18) Imanaka H, Koide H, Shimizu K, Asai T, Kinouchi Shimizu N, Ishikado A, Makino T, Oku N. Chemoprevention of tumor metastasis by liposomal beta-sitosterol intake. *Biol Pharm Bull.* 2008 Mar;31(3):400-4.

19) Sakihama Y, Maeda M, Hashimoto M, Tahara S, Hashidoko Y. Beetroot betalain inhibits peroxynitrite-mediated tyrosine nitration and DNA strand cleavage. *Free Radic Res.* 2011 Nov 17. [Epub ahead of print]

20) Mares-Perlman JA, Fisher AI, Klein R, et al. Lutein and zeaxanthin in the diet and serum and their relation to age-related maculopathy in the third national health and nutrition examination survey. *Am J Epidemiol.* 2001;153(5):424-432.

21) Egert S, Bosy-Westphal A, Seiberl J, Kürbitz C, Settler U, Plachta-Danielzik S, Wagner AE, Frank J, Schrezenmeir J, Rimbach G, Wolffram S, Müller MJ. Quercetin reduces

systolic blood pressure and plasma oxidised low-density lipoprotein concentrations in overweight subjects with a high-cardiovascular disease risk phenotype: a double-blinded, placebo-controlled cross-over study. *Br J Nutr.* 2009 Oct;102(7):1065-74.

22) Sok DE, Cui HS, Kim MR. Isolation and bioactivities of furfuran type lignan compounds from edible plants. *Recent Pat Food Nutr Agric.* 2009 Jan;1(1):87-95.

23) Das S, Tyagi AK, Kaur H, Cancer modulation by glucosinolates: A review *Current Science*, 2000; 79(12)

24) Hayes JD, Kelleher MO, Eggleston IM. The cancer chemopreventive actions of phytochemicals derived from glucosinolates. *Eur J Nutr* 2008 May;47 Suppl 2:73-88.

25) Navarro SL, Li F, Lampe JW. Mechanisms of action of isothiocyanates in cancer chemoprevention: an update. *Food Funct* 2011 Oct 14;2(10):579-87

26) Chao PC, Huang CN, Hsu CC, Yin MC, Guo YR. Association of dietary AGEs with circulating AGEs, glycated LDL, IL-1Ð and MCP-1 levels in type 2 diabetic patients. *Eur J Nutr* 2010; 49(7):429-34

27) Vincent AM, Callaghan BC, Smith AL, Feldman EL. Diabetic neuropathy: cellular mechanisms as therapeutic targets. *Nat Rev Neurol* doi: 10.1038/nrneurol.2011.137, 2011 Sep 13. [Epub ahead of print]

28) http://health.gov/dietaryguidelines/2010.asp

29) Zeidana F, Johnson SKJ, Diamond BJ, David Z, Goolkasianb P. Mindfulness meditation improves cognition: Evidence of brief mental training. *Consciousness and Cognition* 2010;19(2): 597-605

30) Kiecolt-Glaser JK, Christian L, Preston H, Houts CR, Malarkey WB, Emery CF, Glaser R. Stress, Inflammation, and Yoga Practice *Psychosom Med* 2010;72(2): 113

31) Simpson N, Dinges DF. Sleep and Inflammation *Nutrition Reviews* 65(12) s244-252